tele
psychiatry

THE FUTURE
OF MENTAL HEALTH

Robert Plotkin

Editor in Chief - Phil Elmore
http://www.philelmore.com

Consulting Editor - Bob Poole
http://bobpoole.com

Book Design by Jana Rade
http://www.impactstudiosonline.com

Published by Liverpool Press

First Published in 2016 by Liverpool Press – 31 Bryant Drive – Perkasie, PA 18944

First Edition

Copyright ©Robert Plokin
All Rights Reserved

ISBN-13 978-0-9824208-3-6

ISBN-10 0-9824208-3-8

This book is dedicated to all those suffering in silence. It is these people whom we hope to reach. In many ways, I wish this service had been available to my father, who never sought treatment for his mental health issues. In 1974, when I was 10, he committed suicide. He was alone in his thoughts, cornered by the demons he could not speak about. Had he reached out, or had his primary care doctor only possessed the tools needed to assess my father competently, this tragedy might have been avoided.

I therefore dedicate this book to all those patients we want want to reach -- and to all those patients whom we must reach.

Table of Contents

Framing the Problem

I n the last several years, healthcare – particularly *mental healthcare* – has become increasingly prominent in the minds of Americans. Driven by contentious debates about the place ofhealthcare in American lives, not to mention burgeoning shortages of qualified mental healthcare providers, awareness of the problem has outpaced resources devoted to addressing the problem. As the industry works to catch up to that need, and to serve all those who require care, both service providers and the public at large (up to and including insurance companies) are becoming increasingly willing to embrace solutions previously considered "unconventional." Put simply, the market for mental healthcare is expanding, while providers operating in that market are scrambling to evolve fast enough to cover the new ground being opened. At the forefront of this new territory in mental healthcare, forging paths that will in soon become well established, are those providing telemental health generally and telepsychiatry specifically.

This book makes the case for telepsychiatry: Why it is needed, why it works so effectively, and why you should support it. The mainstreaming of telepsychiatry is a process still very much ongoing. This is in some ways surprising, given the results telepsychiatry achieves when it is implemented. Liabilities are few, if any, while the benefits (chief among which are improved logistics and financial savings) are significant. Nonetheless, it is necessary to continue making the case for the widespread implementation and mainstream acceptance of telepsychiatry (and telehealth in general) as the public and private sectors take first small steps, then great strides towards adoption of these remotely provided services.

Public Mental Health in the United States

The mental health problem in the United States continues to worsen. According to the United States government, one in five American adults have experienced a mental health issue. One in ten young people have experienced a major depression, while one in 20 Americans live with a serious mental illness, such as bipolar disorder or schizophrenia. Startling as those numbers are, treatment numbers are far worse:Only

38% of adults with diagnosable mental health problems (and less than 20% of children and adolescents) receive needed treatment.[1]

The raw numbers are just as sobering: The National Alliance of Mental Illness estimates that 61.5 million Americans experience mental illness every year. Almost 15 million of those suffer from major depression, while another 42 million people suffer from anxiety disorders, and almost 10 million have co-occurring mental health and addiction issues.[2] The United States spends $113 billion annually on mental health treatment, which is just less than six percent of the national total (a figure on par with other major industrialized nations).

Most of that money goes to outpatient treatment and prescription drugs – underscoring a shift away from inpatient treatment that began in the 1960s, as centralized institutionalization of the mentally ill fell out of favor. Most painful (and emphasized by the numbers of homeless persons with mental illness) is the fact that Americans simply are not getting the care they require. There are an estimated ninety million Americans living in federally designated "Mental Health Professional Shortage Areas," compared to two thirds that number experiencing shortages of primary care physicians and dentists.[3]

A Brief History of Mental Illness in America

How did we get to this point? How did such a widespread and pervasive problem grow so large so quickly, before steps were taken to address Americans' mental health needs? For most of history, the mentally ill were considered to have something horribly wrong with them – the stigma of which made them social outcasts (and, much less frequently, objects of reverence). By the nineteenth century, it was common practice among industrialized nations to warehouse the mentally ill in frequently deplorable conditions. This began to change with the creation of federally funded state psychiatric hospital. The inpatient care model was notorious for its abuses (the term "bedlam" derives from Bethlem Royal Hospital in London, notorious for the horrible and chaotic conditions in which the mentally ill lived while essentially imprisoned there) and, over the next hundred years, the push for an outpatient model increased.

In 1963, the Community Mental Health Centers Act implemented standards preventing the commission to state psychiatric hospitals of those patients who were not an imminent danger to themselves or others. More than half a million people were institutionalized in the 1950s, but in just thirty years, that number was reduced by 75%. The number of state psychiatric hospital beds fell dramatically as well, by a staggering 94%[4]

The results of widespread deinstitutionalization have been grim. Three to five percent of those with serious mental illness are potentially violent; they are also more than ten times more likely to be the victims of violent crime themselves. The Substance Abuse and Mental Health Services Administration estimates that up to one in four homeless people suffers from some form of severe mental illness.[5] And our national mental health issues do not stem merely from releasing the mentally ill into the wider population, where they often become entangled with the criminal justice system. We are also making the problem larger every day simply by getting better at treating it, making us our own worst enemies where the psychiatric care shortage is concerned.

As the field grows more sophisticated and it becomes possible to diagnose and treat mental health issues with increasing specificity, we naturally redefine the boundaries of the problem outward. For example, diagnoses of autism have increased dramatically in the last several decades. Over the last 45 years, that rate has climbed from 1 in 2,000 children to 1 in 150 children. That increase is due to an expansion of the diagnostic criteria for autism, which now designates patients on a spectrum that includes a broader number of disorders somewhere on that spectrum. It's not that we've seen a dramatic rise in autism among our children; it's that we're diagnosing them more accurately. In the process, though, we've identified an increased need for treatment and thus widened the gap between that need and the number of providers available to address it.[6]

A similar case can be made for many areas of mental health; autism is just one very specific example from among hundreds, if not thousands, of possible mental issues. Yet the stigma of mental illness persists despite the numbers of Americans who are themselves affected by it, either directly or indirectly. Against this backdrop, many Americans do not receive the treatment they require.There are multiple barriers to receiving treatment, two major components of which are accessibility and cost.

Mental Health Professional Shortage Areas

We referred earlier to Mental Health Professional Shortage Areas. This is defined as a geographic area that meets certain criteria. First, the area is, rationally, one where mental health services good be delivered. Second, it must meet certain ratio criteria (such as a population to psychiatrist ratio equal to or greater than 20,000 to 1) or have unusually high needs for mental health services. Mental health professionals in contiguous areas are considered over utilized or excessively distant (or otherwise physically inaccessible). The criteria for a Shortage Area designation are fairly complicated, but those are the broad strokes. In the United States, there are almost 4,000 such shortage areas designated.

Overall, it is estimated that only half of the nation's total mental health treatment needs are being met. The number of practitioners needed simply to remove the Shortage Area designation numbers in the *thousands*. Simply put, there are too few mental health professionals, who live too far away from too many individuals in need of mental health treatment.[7] Mental Health America estimates the ratio of mental health providers to people in the United States at 1 to 790, with only 41% of those with mental illness reporting that they are receiving treatment. This translates to 96.5 million Americans who live in designated Shortage Areas, a number that is up by 5.5 million in just two years.

According to technologist and author Chris Weiss, there are multiple reasons that people do not seek out mental health services even if they do have access to qualified personnel. Cost is a major factor, cited in half of all cases of adults in a 2011 report from the Substance Abuse and Mental Health Administration. But among those patients who could conceivably afford the high cost of care, many simply don't know where to go, or think they don't have the time to go there and be treated. Then too, some patients believe wrongly that they don't need to be treated, or that treatment cannot help them. The stigma associated with mental illness causes them to worry that others will treat them differently if they learn of a mental health diagnosis (which makes concerns about confidentiality a major problem, too). This means the populations most underserved by mental health services are those coping with, or concerned about, one or more of these factors: physical access, cost, convenience, and confidentiality.[8]

The Toll Taken by Untreated Mental Illness

All of this untreated mental illness has costs associated with it. The National Alliance on Mental Illness estimates the hidden costs of untreated mental illness could be as much as $100 billion annually in lost productivity alone. Other hidden costs include those associated with the criminal justice system: those with untreated mental illness tend to act out violently or simply erratically, causing them to be arrested and imprisoned (where they are frequently further victimized). Warehousing our mentally ill in prisons costs money and creates a cycle of crime that, arguably, produces further costs until the person in question is eventually and effectively treated (or simply dies). Suicides, among the top three causes of death for young people and in the top 15 killers of all Americans, could also be prevented by timely application of mental health treatment; up to 90% of suicide victims suffer from mental illness —a fact underscored by the drop in suicide rates in those states mandating mental health coverage for health insurance packages.[9] Less quantifiable, but no less real, are the quality of life issues that could be improved if Americans who require mental health treatment actually receive it. Ignoring this problem, or failing to find new ways to combat it, is hurting us a people, costing us vast sums of money, and resulting in the imprisonment and early deaths of millions of Americans who might, with treatment, lead better lives.

Telepsychiatry is the Solution

There is a solution to all these problems. There are, in fact, multiple solutions, but one among them can address all of these major issues. This solution is telehealth – telepsychiatry, teleEAP, and telemental health services that deliver needed mental health treatment to patients who are located remotely to the provider. This growing, innovative field of treatment is still working toward mainstream acceptance.

While it is seeing great gains, telepsychiatry has further to go before its benefits are fully integrated into modern society.

Telepsychiatry, by its very nature (and thanks to qualities inherent to it), addresses all of fundamental barriers to accessing mental health services: it reduces costs, it increases convenience, it enhances the perception of confidentiality, and it mitigates the logistical problems that might make a provider physically inaccessible. The spread of telepsychiatry thus relieves pressure on the mental health industry while helping patients who need care to get that care. In that way, telepsychiatry alleviates patients' concerns about the cost and implications of the treatment, while making it physically and financially possible for the patients to receive that treatment. If the widespread mental healthcare shortage is to be addressed effectively, it will – it *must*, in fact – be addressed through telepsychiatry.

What is Telepsychiatry?

B efore we continue, we should define some terms. Many of these terms are used interchangeably within the industry, to varying degrees of precision. The first is telepsychiatry itself. Telepsychiatry is applying the field of telemedicine to psychiatry. This means it is the delivery of psychiatric care (diagnosis and treatment) to patients who are located remotely to the service provider using video conferencing technology. Telepsychiatry differs from telemental health in that telepsychiatry is performed by psychiatrists only, while telemental health refers to licensed therapists who provide behavioral health counseling. (This is further differentiated from teleEAP, which we will discuss in the next chapter.) For our purposes in this book, we will use the term telepsychiatry to refer to both psychiatrists and licensed therapists, in that a patient seeking mental health who receives remote treatment will conceivably encounter both of these types of providers (as well as others).

Telepsychiatry is, at its core, extremely simple. Using modern video teleconferencing technology, a provider located remotely to the patient sees, talks to, and listens to the patient (or patients) through the video link. Patients access telepsychiatric care at a supervised location, They aren't simply "dialing in" from their living rooms, though they could, and they are usually referred by their primary care physician if the provider doesn't have a contract with their PCP. Patients thus are typically under the care of a PCP with whom the provider has permission to be in contact. Direct intervention can be undertaken should a patient become distressed.

The goals are simple, too: Telepsychiatric care delivers needed mental healthcare to patients who would not be able to receive them (or who would be disinclined to receive them) if they had to visit a provider in person for face-to-face care. The field has come a long way since the 1960s – and promises, in the coming years, to move forward at a greatly accelerated pace. This has occurred in spite of regulatory and social barriers to the widespread adoption of telemental healthcare.

Some History of Telepsychiatry

In some ways, telepsychiatry simply was not possible until recently. The first telepsychiatry sessions occurred on black and white closed-circuit televisions in the late 1950s and early 1960s. The then primitive technology was used for training, consultation, diagnostic assessment and even group therapy. A few years later, in the late 1960s, a microwave relay was used for the first time to effect a direct consultation at a rural hospital. The term "telepsychiatry" as coined shortly thereafter, in 1973, when adjustable closed-circuit cameras allowed doctors at the Massachusetts General Hospital to treat patients at a nearby airport.[10]

If not for the relatively recent explosion of mobile Internet connectivity, the proliferation of smartphones and tablets, and advances in secure teleconferencing communications, telepsychiatry might have remained relatively rare, incurring thousands of dollars in costs to set up and relegating it to only specialty practices and cases. The modern integration of the Internet and mobile wireless technology has changed all that. Where once, the connection speeds available and the picture quality possible would not have been acceptable, that has changed (and continues to improve). Improve as well are providers' ability to secure those communications in order to achieve HIPAA compliance.[11]

Specialties within telepsychiatry include in-home telepsychiatry (most video technology is encrypted and secure and documentation takes place in a system that is consistent with HIPAA regs), on-demand telepsychiatry (which provides evaluation and treatment on an emergency basis, such as in emergency departments, jails, and substance abuse treatment centers, not to mention mental health facilities), and forensic telepsychiatry (allowing psychiatrists or licensed therapists to treat individuals in correctional facilities, primary care practices, outpatient clinics and similar locations). The Health Insurance Portability and Accountability Act requires certain safeguards for privacy and security be in place for the electronic exchange of medical information, and that includes telepsychiatry. This has led to the creation of specialized videoconferencing methods and HIPAA-compliant technologies.

Legacy Technologies

Legacy technologies in the teleconferencing and telepsychiatry fields include Polycom, a corporation that has been producing videoconferencing equipment since the late

1990s. In the year 2000, the company introduced a desktop video conferencing appliance. Six years later, it was offering an "immersive telepresence solution" and a variety of other high-cost, high-technology videoconferencingtechnologies.[12] Another legacy systems provider is Tandberg, a Norwegian electronics manufacturer acquired by Cisco Systems in 2010. Tandberg's IP-based videoconferencing equipment proved to be Polycom's major competitor in the early 2000s, including (by the middle of the last decade) a desktop videophone. The company's personal videoconferencing system, essentially a dedicated phone with a camera and screen, was introduced in 2008.

The problem with these legacy systems was that they were and are extremely expensive. While such systems make teleconferencing and telepsychiatry possible in specialty and commercial settings, the prohibitive setup costs eliminate such systems from consideration for in-home use. They also constitute a considerable barrier to entry for a psychiatric practice or third-party provider what wishes to establish telepsychiatry services in an underserved market. Stated another way, before the advent of widespread and inexpensive Internet access and teleconferencing equipment, it was simply too expensive, in many cases, to implement telepsychiatry on anything resembling a widespread basis.

Modern Telepsychiatry Technologies

Modern browser-based systems, by contrast, make it extremely easy and inexpensive to set up such services, at least until regulatory compliance is taken into consideration. The typical smartphone, such as an iPhone, has the camera and broadcast capability to convey sound and video at resolutions that are perfectly acceptable. Tablets (such as the iPad), laptop computers, and desktop systems do so commonly. The issue then becomes one, primarily, of security for HIPAA restrictions, rather than the cost or limitations of the technology itself (although bandwidth is still an issue where mobile networks are concerned).

For example, VSee, a proprietary low-bandwidth video chat application, allows users to teleconference at data transfer rates as low as 50 kbit/s (which means real-time video communications are possible over 3G wireless networks). The company introduced a Mac client in 2011 and a secure instant messaging service in 2012. That instant messaging application is so secure, in fact, that it is approved by the United States Congress for use behind the government's firewall.[13]

Another application, doxy.me, is a free, secure telemedicine program that establishes an encrypted, peer-to-peer conduit for the transmission of personal health information between patients and providers. This makes the application HIPAA compliant.[14] Available for computers and mobile devices, the service allows doctors to share their URLs with patients (for example, doxy.me/DrName) and establish secure communications through the Internet. Specifically designed to facilitate "clinical workflow," doxy.me requires no software downloads to work, making it both secure and inexpensive for users.[15]

The development of the WebRTC application programming interface, a set of routines, protocols, and tools for real-time communications over the Internet, supports browser-to-browser applications for voice calling, video chat, and peer to peer file sharing, making it essential for understanding and complying with regulatory policies governing telepsychiatry. This is especially important because those regulations vary from state to state.

The whole point of telepsychiatry, and the benefits derived from it, stems from the ability to deliver psychiatric care to underserved populations at remove from the provider. Underserved populations can exist anywhere, not just rural or remote locations. If there is a lack of providers and it is not possible for those who need care to receive timely scheduled appointments, that market is underserved.Because there are multiple regulations at the federal and state levels, and because there is no single set of federal laws governing telemedicine, it is notoriously difficult to provide telepsychiatric services across state lines – the very thing that makes telepsychiatry of benefit.

The Regulatory Landscape

As contentious as the current regulatory landscape is, it is poised to change... and to improve. The State of Georgia, for example, issued a slate of rules governing telemedicine in 2014, which among other things require an in-person examination prior to telepsychiatric treatment.[16] There are numerous other rules as well. Georgia also now mandates that Licensed Clinical Social Workers, Licensed Professional Counselors, and Licensed Mental Health Counselors receive six hours of training in online counseling. That's just one state in 50; nationwide, telepsychiatry continues to achieve increasing mainstream acceptance – although barriers to its adoption, including legal and regulatory issues, remain.

The Supreme Court recently chose not to hear the case of a veterinarian charged with illegally performing his services via e-mail. Roy Hines, 69, brought his case against the Texas State Board of Veterinary Examiners. At issue was a Texas statute that says a veterinarian may not offer advice through the Internet, or even by phone, unless he first examines the animal in question.

There is some important context here, too: A telemedicine firm, Teladoc, is suing the Texas Medical Board. The issue there is a rule passed by the Board that requires doctors to visit with a patient face-to-face before they can prescribe medication. Teladoc claims the rule violates antitrust laws, and that its purpose is only to place an undue burden on telemedicine companies. The conflict between Teladoc and the Texas Medical Board has been ongoing for several years now. The degree to which a medical board can limit the practice of a telemedicine company hangs in the balance, at least in Texas. That brings us back to Roy Hines' case.

Hines claims that forbidding him to offer his veterinary advice through e-mail is a violation of his Constitutionally protected right to free speech. Where his case gets complicated is in the tricky "intersection of free speech and government licensing of occupations that involve speech," according to journalist Jonah Comstock. Comstock asserts in MobiHealthNews that existing Texas law on the topic is based on a weak precedent. "..While this case isn't directly relevant to the ongoing Teladoc lawsuit with the Texas State Medical Board, it does highlight another legal challenge Teladoc could choose to employ if the antitrust angle doesn't pan out in their favor. And just because the Supreme Court declined to hear the canine version of this case doesn't mean they wouldn't weigh in on a future human version."[17]

The possibility of such a case represents an important tipping point for the future of telepsychiatry. If the benefits of telepsychiatry are to continue accruing to more Americans, legal barriers to service provision MUST be removed. That's a fancy way of saying that if we want to continue helping people, the government must get out of the way and allow service providers using telepsychiatry to provide it. The good news is that telehealth technologies generally are increasing their penetration to the American healthcare market. As other remote technologies achieve acceptance and become commonplace (which we will see in the coming years), acceptance of telepsychiatry will – or should – increase apace.

Mainstreaming Telehealth Technologies

Among the medical technologies already "mainstreaming" are teleradioology (transmission of radiological images from one location to another, allowing physicians and radiologists to compare notes or provide analyses at remove) and telestroke (providing stroke care and exchanging medical data remotely).

Telestroke nicely illustrates the benefits of telemedicine overall. A patient who presents at a rural hospital with stroke symptoms might be out of luck if a qualified doctor with stroke treatment expertise is unavailable. The ER physician, however, can use telemedicine to consult with neurologist located in a more densely populated urban area. That neurologist would be able to access and view CT scans digitally, then advise the ER physician on treatment. This timely access to qualified care saves lives when minutes count —and if it can do this in an ER setting, which is arguably more physically urgent than most counseling and mental healthcare issues, the benefits to telepsychiatry stand to be as great if not greater. With qualified providers in short supply, video teleconferencing technology makes it possible to reach underserved patients while simultaneously making it possible for a single provider to take on a greater patient load. Transit time is eliminated, as are the costs associated with travel, which of course improves the logistics concerned—but it also creates cost savings that are in turn passed on to the very patients the telemedicine services are intended to help.[18]

Interestingly, one of the most active applications for telemedicine in the United States is teledermatology, precisely because advanced communication technologies are well-suited to dermatological diagnoses.[19]

The Clear Choice for Telepsychiatry

Telepsychiatry may be used to reach those populations who are difficult to serve, or who provide greater challenges for service, but this is not always the case. While telepsychiatry is extraordinarily useful for providing care to underserved or physically remote areas, it also increases access to care through cost reduction. A patient who cannot afford psychiatric treatment may be able to afford it at the lower costs achieved through telepsychiatry, in which one provider serves multiple, geographically disparate areas (eliminating travel costs and making it possible for a single provider to serve more patients overall).

The patient base for telepsychiatry includes correctional facilities, emergency departments, school-based programs, primary care practices, outpatient clinics, residential programs, and programs at colleges and universities. A telepsychiatry provider is a board-certified or board eligible psychiatrist who may treat children, adolescents, and adults, and who must be fully credentialed and trained in the videoconferencing technologies utilized. Telepsychiatrists are joined in their efforts by telemental health providers – licensed, master-level clinicians with behavior health experience, usually with a minimum of five years post-licensed and extensive experience in cognitive behavioral therapy and motivational interviewing. They also, typically, have family therapy experience.

Telepsychiatry patients usually receive treatment at clinics and facilities, where supervision is provided (so that help can be offered if patients become distressed) and where regulatory compliance and security protocols can be ensured. Increasingly, though, insurers are paying for in-home psychiatric services, which means patients will have more choices (and greater access to covered care) in the future. Making inroads towards mainstream acceptance with insurance companies is extremely important to telepsychiatry as a field. The insurance industry is more complicated than ever before, but more insurance companies are covering telemedicine services. This bodes well for the industry as a whole and increases access to these services.

Simply put, telepsychiatry gives providers greater choice of personnel while giving patients greater access to care at lower costs. While it is not yet the "delivery system of choice" for psychiatrists and psychologists, it is rapidly becoming so.[20]Telepsychiatry is more convenient, provides a greater perception of security and confidentiality, and allows fewer providers to serve a broader client base. While regulatory and insurance coverage obstacles remain, the limits to telepsychiatry are no longer defined by the technologies involved. Instead, the expansion and mainstream adoption of telepsychiatry is a matter of informing the public – and creating policies, nationally and industry-wide, that support telepsychiatry's many benefits.

What is TeleEAP?

According to the Employee Assistance Trade Association, EAP is an employer-sponsored service designed for personal or family problems, including mental health, substance abuse, various addictions, marital problems, parenting problems, emotional problems, or financial or legal concerns. This is typically a service provided by an employer to the employees, designed to assist employees in getting help for these problems so that they may remain on the job and effective.[21] While EAP was originally focused on substance abuse issues, it is now strongly associated with mental health and counseling as well.

The United States Office of Personnel Management describes EAP as a voluntary, work-based program that offers free and confidential assessments, short-term counseling, referrals, and follow-up services to employees who have personal and/or work-related problems. EAPs address a broad and complex body of issues affecting mental and emotional well-being, such as alcohol and other substance abuse, stress, grief, family problems, and psychological disorders. EAP counselors also work in a consultative role with managers and supervisors to address employee and organizational challenges and needs. Many EAPs are active in helping organizations prevent and cope with workplace violence, trauma, and other emergency response situations.[22]

The primary purpose of EAP in any work setting, then, is both to foster employee well-being and promote positive corporate culture while also reducing costs associated with the loss of productivity that occurs when employees experience mental, emotional, chemical, and financial difficulty.EAP thus fulfills a vital role in ensuring the smooth and efficient operation of any business, regardless of size and the number of employees served.

Arcadian Telepsychiatry Innovated TeleEAP and Changed an Industry

Arcadian Telepsychiatry was at the forefront of applying video conferencing and telepsychiatry methods and techniques to EAP services. It was Arcadian, in fact, that coined the term (and innovated the concept of) TeleEAP. Given that EAP takes place in a work setting (or rather, the process is at least initiated based on an employee's access to EAP), clients for Employee Assistance are both the employees and their employers. TeleEAP programs provide on-demand, expedited assessment, diagnosis, treatment, and disposition of patients in a wide variety of settings, enabling clinicians (typically licensed, master-level counselors experienced with EAP services) to provide short-term clinical counseling and therapy remotely to employees (or *members*, as they are called) through teleconferencing methods (including video and audio).

Numerous mental and emotional issues, such as mild depression, loss, grief, family issues, stress, marital problems, and substance abuse, can be mitigated or treated through counseling services offered by employers in the workplace. Employers may fail to estimate correctly just how costly these issues may be in terms of lost hours of productivity and other factors that affect the bottom line.Only effective treatment, ideally through confidential and accessible Employee Assistance Programs, can prevent or ameliorate these potentially expensive workplace issues.

TeleEAP delivers therapy and short-term clinical counseling to those previously underserved or otherwise reluctant to avail themselves of their EAP programs. It is an excellent tool for combating underutilization of treatment.It also reduces costs both to the employer and the employee in that it provides remote access where direct access would prove too costly or inconvenient.

How TeleEAP Works

The EAP process usually begins when an employee contacts his employers' EAP number or website to inquire about counseling services. This initiates a process wherein the employee is evaluated by a representative for the member's suitability to short-term counseling in a remote setting. A certain number of sessions are authorized by the EAP service as covered by that service and/or employee insurance. (An employee may then have the option of qualifying for more sessions, or paying out of pocket for additional counseling with the same counselor. If the issue is not resolved when the employee's authorized sessions conclude, he or she will be referred back to his or her health insurance provider.)

The benefits of teleEAP compared to more traditional, face-to-face counseling are significant. Remote counseling through videoconferencing makes it possible to provide counseling to previously underserved or unreachable clients.

Qualities specific to TeleEAP make it ideal for reducing or eliminating entirely the barriers to use of EAP programs. These same qualities also make TeleEAP an attractively efficient and cost effective means of fulfilling employees' EAP needs.

Because TeleEAP can reach anywhere that an Internet connection can reach, this delivery system for EAP can serve multiple locations that were previously difficult to reach.These include rural communities dealing with a scarcity of qualified mental health professionals (a problem more common among telemental health providers in general than with TeleEAP providers) and of course residences (as,in some cases, employees may avail themselves of TeleEAP from the comfort of their own homes).

It's important to note that TeleEAP is not synonymous with telepsychiatry. TeleEAP can be conducted remotely with the employee in *any* location, including the employee's home. Until recently, telepsychiatry was conducted with the patient ensconced in a remote treatment facility. (New models have been developed by Arcadian Telepsychiatry in particular that allow safe treatment within the patient's own home. When the patient calls after being referred by his or her doctor, an initial assessment is performed to determine appropriateness for televideo counseling.) The goal is to make sure that personnel are on hand who can respond to patient distress. An employee who utilizes TeleEAP has *already* been evaluated by his EAP representative, who determines his or her suitability for short-term resolution-focused counseling.

The Benefits of TeleEAP

The benefits of TeleEAP are, again, significant. These include increased convenience and improved scheduling logistics, improved cost efficiency, the provision of culturally and ethnically competent providers, greater perception of patient-provider confidentiality, ease of introduction to mental health treatment (and decreased stigma associated with treatment), a therapeutic alliance that is comparable to face-to-face treatment, reduced employer costs, and improved return on employer investment.

Increased Convenience, Immediacy, and Flexibility

Attendant to the nature of accessing any health or wellness service remotely is the flexibility of the medium.In the context of EAP, any tablet or smartphone equipped with HIPAA compliant video conferencing software can be used if the client can find a private area in which to meet virtually with the EAP counselor. This reduces disruption in the workdays of both the client and the provider and allows for greater flexibility in scheduling.This, in turn, makes services faster to access.

The choice of locale is up to the client, which means the client can select those parameters with which he or she is more comfortable. It's also possible for couples and family members to participate in counseling from different locales. This makes it easier to coordinate busy schedules for multiple people, but also increases the comfort factor to include those members who might not participate in counseling if they had to present themselves in person at a provider's office.

This "comfort factor" is an important driver of one of TeleEAP's key benefits. If the member feels he or she is in greater control, he or she will be more comfortable with the process overall and more likely to use the service (both initially and over time). The videoconferencing format is also an essential "leveler," in that it helps reduce the perception of power on the part of the provider. This helps the member to better and more quickly achieve rapport with the provider.

The immediacy of TeleEAP allows for rapid identification and resolution of a member's presenting issues. Fast access, combined with reduced or eliminated travel logistics, means that TeleEAP can reach underserved populations – those who are too far away, physically, to avail themselves of a provider's services, or who are located in shortage areas where wait times for a provider are very long.

Cost-Effectiveness

TeleEAP allows one professional to serve multiple individuals in disparate locations.This reduces overall costs associated with providing the treatment while increasing efficiency for both provider and patient.A provider can simply engage different teleconferences throughout the day from a centralized location or office.Members, in turn, can receive this treatment wherever they happen to be able to access the necessary equipment in relative privacy.The reductions in travel times, the elimination of costly logistics, and the speed with which a provider can service multiple clients makes TeleEAP an incredibly cost-effective alternative to traditional methods of providing treatment to members.

Provision for Culturally and Ethnically Competent Providers

One of the advantages of TeleEAP that may not be immediately apparent is the ability of remote providers to better address *cultural and ethnic competence.* Being able to draw from a larger pool of providers, whose services are accessed remotely by members, allows providers to assign counselors with whom members will be more comfortable, and with whom they can establish a better rapport.

According to the National Center for Biotechnology Information, "In recent years, racial and ethnic disparities in health status and the delivery of healthcare have come to the forefront of healthcare research and policy. These inequities have been documented and summarized in numerous publications... As the evidence of poorer minority health and treatment has accumulated, the emphasis of public policy and research initiatives has shifted from further cataloging the problems to identifying and fostering the implementation of effective strategies to remedy disparities."

One of these solutions is cultural and ethnic competence. "What constitutes cultural competence can vary by healthcare organization, provider-type, organizational and community resources, and patient populations... Culturally competent providers and organizations possess the knowledge, attitude and skills to overcome their own inherent barriers to quality minority care such as biases (e.g. racial/ethnic prejudices, perceived lack of time, and yielding to seemingly overwhelming patient social problems), and service inaccessibility (e.g. inconvenient location, limited appointment availability and lack of care coordination). In addition, culturally competent providers and organizations develop approaches to compensate for patient characteristics that hinder the patient's ability to benefit from healthcare services."[23]

The same features that make TeleEAP ideal for underserved populations in rural areas make it ideal for underserved urban populations, many of which are suffering extreme mental health provider shortages. TeleEAP is also better able to overcome obstacles to care that are endemic to certain demographics and populations (regardless of locale) such as safety and security fears in dangerous neighborhoods (a provider need not be present physically in such an area to provide treatment to residents there), low health literacy among the target population, and lack of resources (such as insurance coverage). Because TeleEAP reduces costs and allows for greater access to the available pool of providers, a better fit can be found for the member at a lower cost overall. That "better fit" includes providing to the member a culturally and ethnically competent provider who can better identify and treat the member's presenting issues.

Patient-Perceived Confidentiality

Because the service is accessed remotely and the patient need never travel to a specific office or medical center, members are much more likely to use the services.The fact that secure encryption is used for video conferencing, and that recordings of the sessions are not made, helps to further reassure patients that their mental health treatment and counseling are discrete, confidential, and private.

Easy Introduction to Mental Health Treatment

Remote treatment allows for a much easier transition to mental health treatment and counseling for most members. The individual may be extremely reluctant to make time in his or her schedule to travel to a provider's office, sit in an unfamiliar setting, and speak to a provider whom the member perceives as intimidating or authoritarian. We've mentioned the "leveling" factor of teleconferencing technology as it pertains to establishing rapport between provider and member. This same quality makes the member more comfortable and makes it easier to transition him or her to mental health treatment after his or her initial assessment.

Decreased Stigma Associated with Mental Health Treatment

The stigma associated with receiving counseling and therapy, as well as concerns about revealing to fellow employees or superiors the need for these services, prevents many from utilizing existing EAPs. TeleEAP eliminates this misperception by allowing the member to conduct his or her business with discretion from the location of his or her choice.

A Therapeutic Alliance Comparable to Face-to-Face Treatment

TeleEAP has been established as comparable to face-to-face counseling in terms of its quality and efficacy. (Arguably, members are sometimes able to establish a rapport with their clinician more quickly thanks to the perceived equality of position when communicating by video teleconference.) Members meet with a highly experienced behavior health clinician virtually. To ensure the member's safety during the session, he or she is asked to provide a physical address as well as the name and telephone number of an emergency contact. This contact is someone to whom the provider would reach out if the need arose during the session.

At present, no studies exist to dispute the efficacy of TeleEAP as compared to face-to-face counseling and therapy programs. The Veterans Administration has, in fact, been using video basedservices to reach underserved and rural areas for almost 20 years.

"A 2008 meta-analysis of 92 studies, for example, found that the differences between Internet-based therapy and face-to-face were not statistically significant (Journal of Technology in Human Services, Vol. 26, No. 2)," writes Amy Novotney. "Similarly, a 2009 review of 148 peer-reviewed publications examining the use of videoconferencing to deliver patient interventions showed high patient satisfaction, moderate to high clinician satisfaction and positive clinical outcomes (Clinical Psychology: Science and Practice, Vol. 16, No. 3).In addition, a 2010 study in the Journal of Clinical Psychiatry (Vol. 71, No. 7) found that videoconferencing can be successful in treating post-traumatic stress disorder. In that study, researchers compared the effectiveness of 12 sessions of anger management therapy delivered via video to in-person delivery of the same treatment to 125 rural combat veterans with PTSD. The researchers found that the video-based anger management therapy was just as effective as the face-to-face care."[24]

Reduced Employer Costs

The National Alliance of Mental Illness estimates that serious mental illness costs 193.2 billion in lost earnings every year. "Lack of treatment impacts more than just productivity," writes Chris Weiss."Many untreated mental health issues lead to an increased likelihood of substance abuse, child abuse, and other domestic problems. The financial ripple effect is much greater than loss of individual productivity, resulting in more services being consumed in other programs."

Take, for example, the issue of depression, an increasingly common malady among American workers. Matt Dunning, reporting for Business Insurance, estimates that employers incur $100 billion annually in direct and indirect costs associated with depression, including as much as $44 billion lost to employee absences and lower productivity.[25]

"Most employers already provide coverage for mental health care under their group benefit plans, as well as access to professional counseling and other resources through employee assistance programs," writes Dunning."However, recent studies indicate that – with the exception of prescription anti-depressant medications – benefits and services aimed at preventing or reducing depression in the workplace are underutilized by employees, which experts say is typically due to a prevailing stigmatization of mental illness in the U.S. that discourages employees from admitting struggles."

The staggering expense of this single workplace issue – and the fact that Dunning highlights underutilization as the primary reason existing EAP programs are not effectively mitigating these direct and indirect costs – underscores the need to address employee access to and use of EAP. When effectively utilized, therapy and short-term clinical counseling can alleviate or even prevent these problems from becoming worse, thereby increasing workplace productivity and reducing lost hours.

Preventive Care and Return on Investment

Most fundamentally, the concept of TeleEAP is one of preventive care. Employers provide members with EAP programs specifically to address mental health issues *before* they become much more serious problems. The old aphorism about an ounce of prevention being worth a pound of cure definitely holds true where mental health is concerned; heading off or preventing serious mental issues or personal problems keeps an employer's workforce happier, healthier, and more productive overall.

Many employers find relatively low utilization of their EAP programs. Steve Albrecht[26], DBA, identifies four primary reasons: First, company stakeholders are not educated about how EAP works, particularly with regard to the confidentiality of the process. Second, employees may feel that a certain stigma attaches to the use of EAP services. They may avoid it because they think they are different or alone, failing to understand that every employee has similar concerns and issues. Third, employees may incorrectly believe they must go through channels in the workplace to avail themselves of EAP, exposing their "issues" to fellow employees and superiors.(In fact, those who use EAP need involve no one from the workplace; they simply contact the provider.)Finally, employees may be unaware of the existence of the EAP program itself.

As we've seen, TeleEAP addresses all of these major issues except the last one (it falls to the employer to properly inform employees of the existence of an EAP program in their workplace). TeleEAP eliminates perceived stigma and increases perceived confidentiality because it can be accessed remotely, in private, without involving fellow employees or the employer directly. By its very nature, TeleEAP is more likely to be accessed by members because it is extremely convenient, up to and including making it easier simply to schedule a session. All of these factors mean an EAP program that makes use of TeleEAP will see increased utilization, which equals better return on the employer's investment in such a program.

Resolution of employee issues produces increased focus, decreased absenteeism, and greater overall workplace morale. Preventive care may also avert potentially serious medical problems and even reduce disability claims. The simple answer is that TeleEAP works, works well, and works *better*, making it the delivery platform of choice for both employers and members who want to get the most benefit and the best value from their EAP programs.

Members TeleEAP Can Help... And Members Better Served Otherwise

TeleEAP is not suitable for everyone (underscoring the importance of the initial member assessment at the beginning of the EAP process), but it is ideally suited to certain types of members, or members with certain specific issues. Remote counseling is well suited to making evaluations for recommendation of a higher level of care. It is also ideally suited to immediately diagnosing the presenting symptoms of depression, anxiety, grief, and Post Traumatic Stress Disorder (PTSD).

For obvious reasons, members suffering from ago-raphobia (an extreme fear of leaving the home or other perceived safe spaces) make good candidates for TeleEAP, and remote videoconference counseling is also suitable for members coping with eating disorders, for crisis debriefing, for counseling of substance abusers who have relapsed, and for verifying medication compliance. Individuals suffering from co-occurring disorders may also benefit from TeleEAP counseling services.

Remote counseling is *not* suitable for patients who are actively suicidal or experiencing homicidal ideation. If they are planning out or intent on committing violence or harm to themselves or others, TeleEAP is not sufficient to their needs. The same is true of couples who are actively experiencing domestic violence. Other patients for whom TeleEAP is not suitable include patients suffering from Alzheimer's or dementia, as they require a greater degree of hands-on, direct care than remote counseling can provide. This is also the case with addicts who are actively abusing moderate to high quantities of alcohol or drugs.

Challenges and Training Solutions

The physical and logistical realities of video teleconferencing technology presents certain challenges to the clinician. This includes the need to engage in relevant safety precautions. When using TeleEAP, for example, an emergency contact must be available within a 25-mile radius of the member being counseled, and that member must provide name and address verification in the event he or she becomes distressed and requires direct intervention. The unique format for teleconferencing counseling raises the issue of "session etiquette" as well; members must receive some form of direction regarding how to use the service and how to get the most out of it.

The very things that make TeleEAP work can prove to be challenging in and of themselves if the member is not fully engaged and cooperative in the process. It's very easy for a disengaged client to simply ignore the provider on the screen, or even feign mechanical difficulties (pretending not to be able to see or hear the provider) in an act of passive aggression or even open hostility. For a member to receive the full benefit of TeleEAP, he or she must cooperate in the process. An individual located remotely from the counselor can refuse to offer this cooperation in extreme cases. Fortunately, because in most cases employees avail themselves of EAP services because they wish it, they tend to cooperate subsequently.

In a similar vein, it can sometimes be difficult to observe body language and read emotional nuances in members when the provider can rely only on what he or she perceives through the teleconferencing link. This requires some adjustment on the part of the service provider. Evolving technologies are making it easier to convey this information, but at the current state of technology, this can still present challenges.

We've mentioned the logistical difficulties regarding state licensure. To say it is not easy to provide mental health care or counseling across state lines is something of an understatement. The requirement to be licensed in the state where treatment occurs presents a unique set of bureaucratic hurdles to surmount.

Finally, one of the technological challenges faced by TeleEAP providers and members is the issue of bandwidth. This is an area where technological advances continue to make it easier and cheaper to transmit ever-larger volumes of data. The next big hurdle faced by the industry is in the area of mobile networks, as Americans increasingly migrate away from desktop computers and toward mobile devices that make use of WiFi and mobile telecom networks.

As in so many things, training may make all the difference when coping with the various challenges to providing TeleEAP. The Telemental Health Institute, for example, offers behavioral telehealth counseling and training, including certificate training packages ranging from introductory courses on telemental health theory to videoconferencing telepractice, legal and ethical issues, advanced clinical telepractice issues, and how-to courses on providing behavioral health and wellness counseling remotely.[27]

Another resource for training is the Online Therapy Institute, which offers training and consultation to mental health practitioners, coaches, and organizations whose focus is in using technology to deliver their services. Training available ranges from post-graduate online training courses to experiential and specialty certification.[28]

Distance Counseling Certification is also available as required by the Center for Credentialing and Education. The various requirements for distance counseling vary by state, and receiving such certification does not mean the provider does not also have to adhere to his or her state's licensure requirements.[29]

How Arcadian Telepsychiatry Changed its Market and Embraced the Future

A rcadian Telepsychiatry is an innovator and business leader in the field of remotely delivering mental health services through technology. This approach is an improvement on the traditional community mental health model of care. As entrenched as the community model is (particularly as it compares and contrasts to a hospital model of institutionalized care), it can be challenging to persuade industry insiders and the public at large to embrace any change from or improvement to the community model. Nonetheless, Arcadian Telepsychiatry made the choice to transition from the community mental health business model to a new model that better provides care to those in need. Embracing this model produces quantifiable benefits to all involved.

Contemporary Arguments for the Community Mental Health Model

The traditional community mental health model is a treatment philosophy based on the social model of psychiatric care that advocates that a comprehensive range of mental health services be readily accessible to all members of the community.[30] Typically, this is defined as the opposite of a hospital-only, institutionalized care model. According to the World Health Organization, "There are no persuasive arguments or data to support a hospital-only approach. Nor is there any scientific evidence that community services alone can provide satisfactory comprehensive care. Instead, the weight of professional opinion and results from available studies support balanced care... [which is] essentially community-based, but hospitals play an important backup role. This means that mental health services are provided in normal community settings close to the population served, and hospital stays are as brief as possible, arranged promptly and employed only when necessary. It is important to coordinate the efforts of various mental health services, whether governmental, nongovernmental or private, and to ensure that the interfaces between them function properly. Cost-effectiveness studies on deinstitutionalization and of community mental health care teams have demonstrated that quality of care is closely related to expenditure. Community-based mental health services generally cost the same as the hospital-based services they replace."[31]

Deficiencies of the Community Mental Health Model

The liabilities of the community mental health model generally center on the negative impacts of *deinstitutionalization* on the American mental health system. "For clients with serious mental illness," write a slate of researchers from Walden University, "learning to live in a community setting poses challenges that are often difficult to overcome. Community mental health agencies must respond to these specific needs, thus **requiring a shift in how services are delivered and how mental health counselors need to be trained**. [emphasis added]"[32]

The contemporary wisdom on deinstitutionalization is that it has resulted in widespread abandonment of individuals who require care – individuals who then find themselves adding to the nation's already pervasive homeless problem or, worse, become entangled in the criminal justice system (where they are then wards of the state whose cost of support falls on the taxpayers, but where they are not necessarily receiving the mental healthcare they require to keep them from committing further criminal acts).

This is mirrored by the experiences of those previously treated, deinstitutionalized patients who, while they may not have entered the criminal justice system, nonetheless relapsed or otherwise deteriorated once left to their own devices within the community (rather than being monitored in an institutional setting). Clearly, *a shift in how services are delivered and how mental health counselors need to be trained* is required – but it cannot be found in any of the old models, which have been tried and which, arguably, have failed to provide necessary improvement.

Changing its Business Model: How Arcadian Telepsychiatry Succeeded

The WHO report underscores the pervasive nature of mental health issues, which account for between 12 and 15% of the total disability in the world. It further asserts that 30% of all years lived are lived with a disability. The key to understanding contemporary attitudes toward the community mental health model lies in the phrase, "quality of care is closely related to expenditure." If community-based mental health services generally cost the same as the institutional services they supplant, where is benefit actually achieved by choosing one model over the other? The answer is that there is no substantive, quantitative change. This points to the reality that Arcadian Telepsychiatry discovered: To actually provide increased benefit and cost savings in the delivery of mental health services, a new business model was required.

Arcadian Telepsychiatry provides psychiatrists and therapists throughteleconferencing to those in need in a **Business to Business to Consumer** format. This is opposed to, and improvement on, the previous community mental health business model which, while it provides steady revenue, offers slim margins and provides care largely to Medicaid recipients. Nonetheless, Arcadian believes strongly in the need to serve all individuals regardless of income level. By moving our model away from community mental health centers, that business model has advanced and matured, allowing us to treat individuals in community settings while also propelling our business forward to reach a broader base of those in need of service.Arcadian's large network of psychiatrists and therapists serves clients in 40 states. The company has cultivated relationships with large insurance companies as well as companies that provide employee assistance program benefits services to employers.

In this way, Arcadian's improved business model uses telemedicine (specifically, telepsychiatry and teleEAP) in the narrow context of behavioral health. This widens access to behavioral healthcare and levels the playing field between rural and urban areas. No longer does location determine access to care. Further, thanks to the cost savings produced by using remote services instead of in-person, face-to-face services, mental healthcare within our business model is provided to a greater number of clients at lower prices, increasing access to needed care among those who require it.

Arcadian is, in fact, a leader in the United States in offering professional mental health services through the use of state-of-the-art video conferencing technology.The company customizes its services to its clients goals. Those clients are health systems and primary care practices, which enroll in commercial insurances for direct reimbursement from the insurance company, and EAP services and corporations requiring EAP services, which offer either fee-for-service or per-member-per-month pricing models.

This is nothing short of a new digital health strategy, which incorporates digital methods (including evaluation and even alcohol assessments) while incorporating digital cognitive behavioral tools to better serve remotely the needs of the clients so reached. Arcadian Telepsychiatry's clinicians support both assessment and cognitive behavioral therapy programs. The mental health professionals working with Arcadian are licensed in the states where clients (members) reside and are supervised by experienced clinical directors. Arcadian has also worked diligently to simplify the technological interface, making the video conferencing aspect as simple and effective as possible.

Access, Access, Access: Why Arcadian Succeeded

The opportunities to identify and secure contracts in such a market, following this business-to-business-to-consumer model, are numerous. Recruiting and finding businesses that require EAP and mental health services is part and parcel of the model. The reason Arcadian succeeded, however, is as simple as it is integral to Arcadian's mission: Improved access.

Imagine that you could save time and money by not driving to get to your professional mental health care service provider. Where ever you are, nationwide, you can connect online instead. Live audio and video feeds give you the personal, one-on-one attention you deserve. The service is discreet, secure, convenient, and costs less than can be provided by the traditional community mental health model. It is, in this way, truly innovative but – much more importantly – it represents substance improvement on the old model in way that gets care to those previously underserved.

If you are a licensed psychiatrist in any state working with Arcadian Telepsychiatry, you can see patients without leaving your office – no matter where it is located. Arcadian encourages qualified mental health professionals to join its network and reach out to serve underserved populations, at lower cost and with greater scheduling flexibility.

How It Works

As we've said, Arcadian's is a business-to-business-to-consumer business model. The company contracts with primary care practices, physicians' groups, health systems, and emergency room departments. It also contracts with insurance companies directly to reach those clients in need of service. Reimbursement procedures vary by state, but accessing services through technology makes the process extremely cost-effective. This includes, increasingly, at-home telepsychiatry, on-demand telepsychiatry, and scheduled visits.

Other Telemedicine and Telepsychiatry Providers

There are multiple firms working in the telemedicine and telepsychiatry fields in the United States today. These include telemedicine companies Teladoc, Doctor on Demand, American Well, and MDLive. Telepsychiatry companies operating today include JSA Health, Forefront Telecare, FarPsych, One-DocWay (recently acquired by Genoa Pharma), ePsychiatry, and of course Arcadian Telepsychiatry.

Teladoc allows users who sign up for an account to talk to a doctor on demand, by phone or video consultation. The site claims that physician response time is less than ten minutes, and prescriptions from your televised doctor can be transmitted to the pharmacy of your choice. Overwhelmingly, patients of Teladoc report that their televised doctor resolved their issue. Teladoc physicians update the patient's HIPAA-compliant electronic health record based on the consultation, and charges are made directly to the patient's credit card on file.[33]

Doctor on Demand is a similar service that allows physicians, psychologists, and lactation consultants to provide focused care through video teleconferencing, diagnosing issues and providing effective treatment plans. Clients pay per visit and incur no other fees; cost varies depending on the length of the session. As is typical with telemedicine services, Doctor on Demand's professionals provide services through the platform that Doctor on Demand provides, but the company itself does not provide healthcare services.[34]Other comparable services include American Well[35] and MDLive.[36]

Of these firms, Teladoc is the only publicly traded company. Teladoc is also, as we mentioned previously, suing the Texas Medical Board to dispute a state regulation requiring doctors to visit with a patient face-to-face before they can prescribe medication. MDLive, meanwhile, recently raised $50 million of new funding in an investment deal, enabling the company to continue expanding and to reach its vision of building a fully integrated, end-to-end virtual health system. MDLive's vice chairman of the board of directors, formerly a CEO of Pepsi and Apple, commented specifically on the need for "transformative change" in the American healthcare system, citing access, quality, and cost as healthcare's greatest challenges.[37]

Competing telepsychiatry companies include JSA Health, which provides psychiatric care to emergency departments, communityhealth clinics, educational institutions, and correctional facilities.[38] Its primary focus is emergency rooms. There is also Forefront Telecare, which links specialists to rural and under-served healthcare facilities (focusing most prominently on nursing homes).[39]The aptly named e-Psychiatry, meanwhile, provides mental health clinics, hospitals, employers, and health plans with a means to connect with qualified psychiatrists and mental health professionals.[40]

OneDocWay, which was acquired by Genoa Pharma in 2015, focuses on community mental health centers. "Many of the Community Mental Health Centers that work with Genoa," wrote Fred Pennic at the time of the acquisition, "are facing increased demand for support as they strive to improve access to care for the communities they serve. One significant barrier to fulfilling that mission is the nationwide psychiatry shortage. Genoa is committed to pioneering solutions that can add value to its relationships and improve patient care. Telepsychiatry provides an innovative solution to the gaps in supply and demand for mental health services, including psychiatrist availability."[41]

Arcadian Telepsychiatry is the Future of Mental Healthcare in the United States

Among all these competitors, and industry-wide, Arcadian Telepsychiatry is uniquely positioned, thanks to its innovative business model, to address the needs of a changing market while reaching the most clients through business providers.

The merits of telepsychiatry are not simply obvious; they are being proven out day after day by the benefits telepsychiatry achieves. Using video conferencing to bring mental health professionals to underserved populations, and to the public at large at reduced cost and with increased convenience, flexibility, and perceived confidentiality, improves access and quality of care while reducing the burden on society when it comes to funding these services. Telepsychiatry is also the logical way to address a nationwide shortage of providers, allowing psychiatrists to treat more patients over a larger area and to reach people for whom a qualified professional was not previously accessible.

For these reasons, telepsychiatry continues to gain greater mainstream acceptance. The trend, industry wide, is toward remote provision of services, not away from it. The telehealth model, and specifically Arcadian Telepsychiatry's business model, is the future of mental healthcare in the United States.

Why Telepsychiatry Matters to Your Health System or Behavioral Health Program

S o, why does telepsychiatry matter to you? What benefits does it offer to your health system or behavioral health program? The answers are simple and, quite frankly, should now be obvious: telepsychiatry reduces cost while increasing access. Telepsychiatry is also critical to integrating mental health with primary care, a model advocated by the World Health Organization.

The Triple AIM Initiative

A critical factor within the mental health industry for health systems and Accountable Care Organizations (ACOs) is the Triple AIM initiative. Triple AIM is "a framework developed by the Institute for Healthcare Improvement that describes an approach to optimizing health system performance."[42] According to the IHI itself, in the majority of healthcare settings, "no one is accountable for all three dimensions of the IHI Triple Aim. For the health of our communities, for the health of our school systems, and for the health of all our patients, we need to address all three of the Triple Aim dimensions at the same time."[43] Those three dimensions, as designated by the IHI, are population health, experience of care, and per-capita cost.

- **Improved population health:** Arcadian Telepsychiatry uses the BIOTRENDS digital assessment tool to assess patients and determine appropriate means and methods of care. For example, BIOTRENDS can be used to assess a patient with diabetes for signs of depression. Using the technologies and methods available to us, Arcadian seeks to improve the overall population health of those needing mental health treatment in the United States by providing more qualified care to populations previously underserved.

- **Improved care experience:** – Telepsychiatry is, by definition, a means of improving the care experience. Not only does it provide care to those who need it (many of whom would not be able to receive necessary care without remote access), but it does so with greater convenience and flexibility. Patients who receive remote care report a greater perception of confidentiality (even though their confidentiality is protected regardless) and may also be faster to achieve rapport with their remote care providers.

- **Reduced per capita costs:** Telepsychiatry also, by its nature, reduces costs by eliminating costly logistics. It also keeps patients out of emergency departments by offering preventive care through population management and improved access to care. All of these factors contribute to overall cost reduction.

Telepsychiatry is well positioned to address the Triple AIM initiative. For that reason, it is critical to your health system or behavioral health program. The benefits of implementing a telepsychiatry infrastructure are both demonstrable and proven.

Integration with Primary Care

The National Center for Biotechnology Information defines mental health in the context of primary care as integrating mental health services with essential healthcare. If primary healthcare is based on the needs of the population, decentralized, and requires the active participation of the community and the family, then mental healthcare involves diagnosing and treating people with mental disorders. This includes "putting in place strategies to prevent mental disorders and ensuring that primary healthcare workers are able to apply key psychosocial and behavioral science skills, for example, interviewing, counseling and interpersonal skills, in their day to day work in order to improve overall health outcomes in primary healthcare."

The integration of primary mental health services are, according to the NCBI, "complementary with tertiary and secondary level mental health services... e.g. general hospital services (short stay wards, and consultation-liaison services to other medical departments), which can manage acute episodes of mental illness quite well but do not provide a solution for people with chronic disorders who end up in the admission–discharge–admission (revolving door syndrome) unless backed up by comprehensive primary healthcare services or community services."[44]

There is undoubtedly social stigma attached to mental health services, including the vast number of mental health services provided on an outpatient basis. Integrating mental healthcare with primary healthcare services reduces this stigma by making mental health treatment part and parcel of the general, primary healthcare the individual already needs and seeks. Because primary healthcare providers are more accessible than specialized, standalone mental health services, they are also more available. "Integrated care helps to improve access to mental health services and treatment of co-morbid physical conditions," writes the NCBI. (Mental health conditions frequently accompany life-threatening chronic or terminal illnesses, which has "serious implications for the identification, treatment and rehabilitation of affected individuals. When primary healthcare workers have received some mental health training they can attend to the physical health needs of people with mental disorders as well as the mental health needs of those suffering from infectious and chronic diseases," leading to better health outcomes.

The HEDIS Metric

The overwhelming majority of America's health plans use the HEDIS metric to measure care and performance in healthcare services.[45]HEDIS comprises scores of measurements across multiple domains of care. Among these are...

- Follow-up after hospitalization for mental healthcare
- Antidepressant medication management
- Diabetes screening for those with schizophrenia or bipolar disorder who are using antipsychotic medications
- Diabetes monitoring for people with diabetes and schizophrenia
- Cardiovascular monitoring for those with cardiovascular disease and schizophrenia
- Adherence to antipsychotic medications for individuals with schizophrenia

Metrics of this type not only put a quantitative face on mental healthcare and its holistic connection to physiological health, but they make it possible to measure success as patients are treated as whole people, with the mind-body connection as a primary concern rather than as an often-ignored afterthought. The push to integrate mental health services with primary care is one of the World Health Organization's recommendations for this reason. It is a laudable goal, worthy of both exploration and investment.

Central to making mental healthcare services more accessible—not to mention integrating them with existing primary care infrastructure—are remote services. Telepsychiatry, because it is delivered remotely through videoconferencing equipment, can be readily integrated into most—if not all—primary care settings. This improves service, provides more holistic mental and physical healthcare, and fulfills the WHO's recommendations for improving the quality of care populations receive.

As telepsychiatry specifically and telehealth generally continue to gain mainstream acceptance, their utility will drive that acceptance. The greater accessibility and lower cost of remote mental health services represent both immediate gains and long-term advantages. They also address chronic shortages of qualified providers. Taken as a whole, these factors would seem to spell the inevitability of telepsychiatry in primary care settings.

How Telepsychiatry Saves Money

Remote teleconference access to mental health services allows one qualified professional to serve multiple individuals in disparate locations.This eliminates the logistics of traveling from location to location, eliminates security concerns associated with some locales or venues (such as in correctional facilities), and allows professionals to focus on providing care rather than simply getting from setting to setting (or, conversely, allows patients to focus on their treatment without worrying about making extra time for an appointment and then getting to the physical location). Providers can work from the comfort of their own offices as they prefer and need never worry about how accessible their location might be to their client base. This further eliminates the need to create satellite offices or to position office locations in areas that may not be convenient to the provider's home.

All of these factors reduce overall costs associated with providing the treatment while increasing efficiency for both provider and patient.A provider can simply engage different teleconferences throughout the day from a centralized location or office.Members, in turn, can receive this treatment wherever they happen to be able to access the necessary equipment in relative privacy (depending on whether they must do so from a supervised clinic to comply with HIPAA guidelines and treatment requirements).The reductions in travel times, the elimination of costly logistics, and the speed with which a provider can service multiple clients makes telepsychiatry an incredibly cost-effective alternative to traditional methods of behavior health treatment. These cost savings can be passed on from providers to members in order to make services more accessible.

How Telepsychiatry Improves Service

The reduction in cost itself makes treatment more accessible to a wider population by reducing its price. Telepsychiatry service further benefits the client because it is more convenient, making scheduling easier. Notably, telepsychiatry makes it easier to provide the client with a culturally and ethnically competent provider with whom he or she can build a greater rapport. This is a direct result of telepsychiatry's ability to connect the patient remotely to a broader base of providers than to whom the client would have access in a face-to-face setting. (As we've discussed, it also may mean the difference between having access to a provider *at all*, or suffering long wait times that are driven by shortages of qualified providers.)

Improved service is further achieved through the enhanced perception of confidentiality. Clients may feel much more comfortable accessing mental health services remotely because they feel more "hidden" in doing so. While this is technically untrue, it is a beneficial fiction, in that anything that gives the client faith in what are already discreet, HIPAA compliant and confidential treatment resources will encourage that client to engage in the necessary treatment. The result is a decreased stigma associated with treatment, all while establishing a therapeutic alliance that is comparable to face-to-face treatment.

The flexibility of the videoconferencing medium reduces disruption in the client's workday, which itself improves flexibility in scheduling and makes services faster to access. Depending on the service (such as teleEAP versus telepsychiatry) the choice of locale is up to the client, which means the client can select those parameters with which he or she is more comfortable. It's also possible for couples and family members to participate in counseling from different locales. This makes it easier to coordinate busy schedules for multiple people, but also increases the comfort factor to include those members who might not participate in counseling if they had to present themselves in person at a provider's office.

The immediacy of telepsychiatry, like teleEAP, allows for rapid identification and resolution of a member's presenting issues. Fast access, combined with reduced or eliminated travel logistics, means that these remote services can reach underserved populations. More importantly, the flexibility and speed with which telepsychiatry can be delivered to the client compared to traditional, face-to-face psychiatry, results in both improved *perception* of the service as well as *quantifiable* improvement in how fast the service reaches the patient. This improvement is critical if we are to improve a troubled healthcare system known for its high cost, barriers to access, and reluctance to embrace certain new technologies that could have immeasurable benefits to the public.

Telepsychiatry's Success with Veterans

Treatment of mental health issues among American veterans has been of ever greater concern in the last several years, as the industry grapples with effective ways to treat PTSD and veterans themselves contend with long wait times for medical treatment through the Department of Veterans Affairs. Finding ways to serve those veterans' needs more thoroughly and more quickly helps solve at least one dimension of this very profound problem. Apply telepsychiatry to veterans' healthcare has produced significant gains for this population of patients.

A study by the National Center for PTSD found that telemental health practices produced substantial benefits for Veterans suffering from Post Traumatic Stress Disorder. "The major benefit of telemental health," reads the study, "is that it eliminates travel that may be disruptive or costly. In addition, telemental health is a useful tool in situations, such as in correctional and forensic settings, where it is difficult to transport the patient to a clinician. Telemental health also allows mental health providers to consult with or provide supervision to one another. ...Findings from pilot data of a PTSD psychoeducation and coping skills group suggest that the Veterans, the clinic staff, and the remote clinician all viewed the VTC treatment as helpful. A comparison of the VTC group to an in-person control group in this study revealed no significant difference between the two groups on measures of satisfaction and information retention."[46] In other words, telepsychiatry, with all its benefits in terms of schedule flexibility, immediacy, and reduced cost, was found to be just as beneficial as in-person therapy for Post Traumatic Stress Disorder.

The Department of Veterans Affairs has released its own statistics, which cover over 690,000 veterans served in Fiscal Year 2014 (more than 2 million virtual visits were scheduled during that period). Consider that carefully: The VA served nearly 700,000 veterans during the 2014 fiscal year, which is about 12 percent of the total VA healthcare population. Those 2 million telehealth visits allowed roughly 55 percent of veterans in rural areas, who have limited access to VA healthcare, to nonetheless receive that needed care. The VA offers more than 44 clinical specialties to Veterans through its telehealth programs (such as teleaudiology, which addresses the large population of veterans who have suffered hearing loss). Telehealth generally, and telepsychiatry specifically, is thus a proven, statistically supportable fact.[47]

Cognitive Behavioral Therapy

Cognitive behavioral therapy (CBT) is a form of psychotherapy originally designed to treat depression. It is now used for a variety of mental problems, and works to solve those problems while changing unhelpful thinking and behavior.[48] Given the nature of CBT, it would seem to be an excellent fit for telepsychiatry. After all, it is nothing more or less than the client talking with the therapist and redefining his or her way of thinking about problems and issues. As it turns out, studies have demonstrated there is no difference in the efficacy or client satisfaction associated with CBT received through one-on-one, in-person therapy versus CBT received through telepsychiatry.

A systematic review of telepsychiatry and CBT published in 2010 concluded that there is"insufficient scientific evidence regarding the effectiveness of telepsychiatry in the management of mental illness, and more research is needed to further evaluate its efficiency. However, there is a strong hypothesis that videoconference-based treatment obtains the same results as face-to-face therapy and that telepsychiatry is a useful alternative when face-to-face therapy is not possible." The study also said that there "were no statistically significant differences between study groups for symptoms, quality of life, and patient satisfaction."[49]

This brings us back to veterans and CBT: The National Center for PTSD reports that a 12-session anger management therapy delivered to a group of patients was compared in a randomized clinical trial to see if using video conferencing technology had any effect on the efficacy of the cognitive behavioral therapy as compared to in-person treatment. "Secondary analyses of the outcomes of this trial indicated that the use of [video conferencing technology] does not affect group therapy process or therapist adherence to a manualized cognitive behavioral therapy protocol."

Dialectical Behavior Therapy

Dialectical Behavior Therapy (DBT) is a cognitive behavioral treatment originally developed to treat chronically suicidal individuals diagnosed with borderline personality disorder. It is considered the "gold standard" of psychological treatment for such patients. Can DBT be delivered through telepsychiatry? Normally, actively suicidal individuals would not be good candidates for remote therapy, but one study of telepsychiatry among incarcerated youth found that it was an excellent solution to the problem of helping a traditionally underserved population (one in which numerous psychiatric disorders, including those treatable with DBT, are present).

Interactive video conferencing was used to connect a minimum security correctional facility with a regional telemedicine program. Clinical records were then reviewed to examine utilization, demographics, diagnoses, pharmacotherapy, and patient satisfaction. The study concluded that telepsychiatry "can successfully deliver services to incarcerated adolescents with a wide range of psychiatric needs. A patient-centered approach that directly assesses adolescents satisfaction is recommended to ensure youths' optimal involvement in needed services."[50]

Exposure Therapy

Exposure therapy is a technique in behavior therapy used to treat anxiety disorders. It involves the exposure of the patient to the feared object or context without any danger, in order to overcome their anxiety.[51] This is significant because anxiety disorders are under-diagnosed and undertreated in primary care. Only a third of patients diagnosed with anxiety receive counseling for the condition, and only a quarter of these people receive counseling from a mental health professional. One in ten of these patients received treatment specific to anxiety disorders.[52]

Telepsychiatry is ideal for presenting exposure therapy specifically, and treatment for anxiety disorders generally. The client can receive treatment at remove from the provider and thus feel more "safe," with his or her comfort level at the highest it is possible to achieve. In exposure therapy, exposure to the anxiety-producing condition can be as simple as a picture on a screen, which is as safe and unthreatening as such exposure gets.

A pilot study of prolonged exposure therapy for PTSD delivered through telehealth technology, conducted in 2010, concluded that telepsychiatry produced "large statistically significantdecreases in self-reported pathology for veterans treated with [prolonged exposure therapy] via telehealth technology. Preliminary resultssupport the feasibility and safety of the modality."[53] That's an elaborate way of saying that the exposure therapy, delivered through telepsychiatry, works, and works well.

Behavior Modification

Behavior modification is the term used for changing behavior to increase or decrease its frequency, altering an individual's reactions to stimuli through positive and negative reinforcement of adaptive behavior.[54] A study published in 2007 in the journal Behavior Modification looked specifically at behavior modification and "manualized cognitive behavioral therapy" for PTSD delivered through videoconferencing technology. "Results from this study," write the researchers, "indicate therapist competence and adherence to a manualized group cognitive-behavioral psychotherapy are similar whether the treatment is delivered via [telepsychiatry] or the traditional means... No statistically significant differences in adherence were found in competence... with more favorable ratings on this item for the [telepsychiatry] condition. These findings suggest that mental health services can be delivered via a telehealth application in a competent manner. Of particular importance is the finding that therapist ratings were identical on items assessing "rapport" and "empathy," which are considered critical components of a successful psychotherapy intervention. [emphasis added]"[55]

The conclusion, in this case, is clear: Not only can behavior modification be delivered through telepsychiatry, but patients actually indicated they found their therapist *more* competent when using telepsychiatry than they did when receiving therapy face-to-face in a traditional setting.

Psychoeducation

Psychoeducation is education offered to individuals with some mental health problem that helps to empower the patient to deal positively with the condition. It is common in treating schizophrenia, depression, anxiety disorders, eating disorders, and personality disorders. Psychoeducation, too, can be delivered through telepsychiatry.

According to the National Center for PTSD, "Therapy provided over the Internet has been among the most controversial applications of telemental health services." The report cites a controlled trial "in which they provided psychoeducation, screening, and a protocol-driven treatment for people suffering from PTSD and grief via the Internet. More than

50 percent of the treated participants in this study showed reliable change and clinically significant improvement. The largest changes were seen in measures of depression and avoidance. Although it is too early to recommend web-based delivery of services, it is likely that the Internet will be increasingly used to supplement face-to-face care."[56]

This means the veterans given psychoeducation through telepsychiatry showed improvement more than half the time. Even if this rate compared unfavorably to in-person psychoeducation, the ease with which such treatment is offered through the Internet indicates it is better to try it than not.

Motivational Interviewing

Motivational interviewing is an attempt to engage the patient's intrinsic motivation in order to change behavior in a goal-oriented, client-centered manner. It helps patients to explore and resolve their own ambivalence toward things they need to change in their lives.[57] A trial by BioMed Central, for example, declared intent to study motivational interviewing for diabetes patient education and support, delivered remotely (in this case, by telephone). "There is increasing interest in developing peer-led and 'expert patient'-type interventions, particularly to meet the support and informational needs of those with long term conditions, leading to improved clinical outcomes, and pressure relief on mainstream health services," reads the study. "There is also increasing interest in telephone support, due to its greater accessibility and potential availability than face to face provided support. ...The hypotheses to be tested in this study are that telecare motivational interviewing will be acceptable to patients and primary care health professionals; will be associated with improved social and psychological status; healthier lifestyle choices; and enhanced satisfaction with care."[58]

Interesting as that sounds, can telepsychiatry be used to deliver motivational interviewing that results in positive change for clients? A study at the University of Colorado looked at the effects of telephone counseling on antipsychotic adherence and emergency department utilization. Its objective was to determine whether a specific telehealth nursing program could reduce emergency department utilization and improve adherence among Medicaid health plan members with serious and persistent mental illness.

The conclusion? "Cognitive-behavioral and motivational-interviewing techniques can improve antipsychotic medication adherence. Telehealth may be a useful strategy for disseminating these evidence-based techniques. Lessons learned included the importance of real-time referral data, a need to address polypharmacy, and a need to overcome contact difficulties resulting from disease processes and "unknown caller" IDs. Despite these difficulties, using a disease management model, the program was feasible, and the reduced number of ED visits indicated potential cost-effectiveness."[59]

Yet again, the study proved the viability of a telehealth platform in delivering these services. While there were some practical considerations, these paled in comparison to the benefits produced.

Problem Solving Therapy

Problem-solving therapy is a cognitive-behavioral intervention used to treat depression. It can help teach you to manage the various stressors in your life that can interact to cause or worsen depression.[60] The question we ask, yet again, is whether this type of therapy can be delivered through telepsychiatry. The results we again produce are a resounding yes.

A 2014 study called "Telehealth Problem-Solving Therapy for Depressed Low-Income Homebound Older Adults: Acceptance and Preliminary Efficacy" evaluated the acceptance and effectiveness of in-home therapy for older shut-ins suffering from depression.The Treatment Evaluation Inventory score, which was the means of measuring the effectiveness of the therapy, was slightly *higher* among the patients who received telepsychiatry. "Despite their initial skepticism, almost all participants had extremely positive attitudes toward tele-PST at 12-week follow-up. Tele-PST also appears to be an efficacious treatment modality for depressed homebound older adults and to have significant potential to facilitate their access to treatment."[61]

The Path Forward Is Clear

In every instance where telepsychiatry is appropriate for treatment, it succeeds. Results range from no difference as compared to in-person, traditional therapy, to improved perception and success rates among clients for services rendered remotely rather than in person. This is a profound statement concerning the feasibility of telepsychiatry and its place in the future of the mental health field. Patients actually seem to *prefer* remotely provided services, and if they do not prefer them, they at least perceive no difference in the efficacy of these services compared to traditional methods of treatment.

Strategies for Success

Telehealth programs are not all created equal. Arcadian Telepsychiatry has, over time, identified a number of best practices for telemental health services that produce the best possible opportunities for successful outcomes. While the scope of such practices might encompass a book all by themselves, we will outline them briefly here. In so doing, we hope to better equip both providers and clients (from individual members to employers and service providers) with a plan for moving forward toward telepsychiatry, teleEAP, and telehealth solutions.

Explain What to Expect

Client comfort is the key to success in the most general sense with telemental health. A client who is anxious, intimidated, or otherwise uncomfortable will find it more difficult to engage with the provider (the clinician) or to cooperate in his or her own treatment. One of the best ways to increase client comfort is to explain to the member what to expect from the process. Patients should be walked through the process from start to finish, including necessary steps for qualifying for more sessions if they are using teleEAP. Security protocols, use of the video teleconferencing equipment, and any etiquette considerations for the communications between provider and client should also be covered.

Explaining what to expect also enhances the leveling effect that takes place when a client receives treatment through a teleconferencing link. The perception of authority on the part of the provider is mitigated, and the client, feeling more of a sense of equality between him- or herself and the provider, will more quickly build rapport with the provider. This helps to maintain both the efficacy of the treatment, but also keep the client engaged so that sessions are not missed and needed counseling is not ignored.

The Clinician Must Be Qualified and Culturally Competent

Cultural competence on the part of the clinician should never be ignored. Given that it is possible to select a clinician from among a wider pool of potential counselors, that clinician should always be selected with cultural competence in mind. Does that clinician possess the knowledge, attitude, and skills to overcome their own inherent barriers to quality minority care? Does he or she have any biases (e.g. racial/ethnic prejudices, perceived lack of time, and yielding to seemingly overwhelming patient social problems) that should be addressed, and have these been addressed through appropriate training? Is service inaccessibility an issue?

A culturally competent clinician will develop a better rapport with the patient, thus keeping the patient more engaged. Cultural touchstones may also help clinician and provider to overcome the patients' innate reluctance to deal with his or her issues. The more common ground shared by the provider and by the client, the easier it will be for the two of them to have productive sessions that actually produced the desired outcomes.

Stated another way, selecting clinicians who are not culturally and ethnically competent will quickly doom the clinical relationship. It is too easy for the client simply to turn away or push a button and end the session. To keep clients engaged, this cultural sensitivity must always be factored into the selection of treatment provider.

Camera Placement and Lighting Must Be Appropriate to Building Rapport

Practical considerations must not be ignored when preparing for the work of a counseling session through teleEAP or tele-psychiatry. If the lighting is poor, the clinician will not be able to see the patient adequately in order to read body language, posture, and other nonverbal cues, up to and including immi-nent emotional distress. The clinician must be able to see the patient, and must be able to see the appropriate amount of the patient's face and upper body, in order both to establish rapport and also to provide appropriate treatment and feed-back. The same is true if the camera is positioned poorly so that one or the other party cannot adequately see each other. Poor camera placement or poor lighting can make both the provider and the client frustrated, leading to unproductive sessions or even sessions that the client quits in anger or disappointment.

Too much light may be just as problematic as too little light. If the patient is receiving telepsychiatry at a remote facility with supervision on hand, it may be the case that lighting has been set up for the clinician's benefit that the patient finds uncomfortably bright. We want to avoid the perception that the patient is being "interrogated" at all costs, and of course a client who is uncomfortable is less likely to achieve success in the course of the session. While walking a client through what to expect from the sessions, therefore, it's a good time to check on lighting, microphone sound levels, transmission bandwidth and quality, and any other practical factors that might affect the session.

That actually brings us to the subject of backup systems and technology problems.

Avoiding Technology Problems and Disruptions

Teleconferencing systems and programs are used throughout the business world, and include video/audio programs that allow users to share computer desktops, trade files, and teleconference multiple individuals at disparate locations. There is not a person alive who has sat through such meetings who has not experienced technical difficulties, sometimes repeatedly, as the meeting organizer tries to get everyone on the call or video conference set up and working. Often, time is wasted setting up these meetings, reducing the efficiency of the meeting and frustrating or angering the attendees.

The same is absolutely true of teleconferencing for teleEAP and telepsychiatry. You cannot afford to experience repeated technical difficulties while also trying to engage with a client. Those problems will disrupt the session, waste the time scheduled for the session, and frustrate the client in a way that could cause him or her to disengage.

Likewise, when a session is going well and the client and provider are achieving results, very little is more disruptive to that process than losing the connection between the two, or otherwise experiencing a problem (like video that is too choppy, or audio that is too quiet). For this reason, a telemental health provider should always have backup systems in place, or at the very least a backup procedure (such as continuing the session by secure telephone connection) should be in place. This minimizes disruption from inevitable technology failures. But simply having a backup plan in place is not enough. That backup plan must be adequately communicated to both providers and clients so that both know what to expect, and how to proceed, in the event of a failure of the teleconferencing infrastructure.

To that same end, the risks and benefits of the video service should be discussed – not just at the outset of treatment, but also over time in the context of the therapeutic relationship. Just as it is sometimes difficult for an observer to remove himself from a scientific experiment in order to achieve true scientific objectivity and therefore objective results, it may be difficult for the provider and the client to remove from the context of their therapeutic relationship the technology that both separates them and unites them. This is why discussing the use of that technology – the advantages it provides, as well as the limitations it imposes on the therapeutic interaction – should be discussed in an ongoing way, to remind both provider and client of the need to attend to this ongoing issue.

The Client Should Be Aware of Other Treatment Options in the Community if they Exist

Any basic understanding of medical ethics demands that a patient who might have treatment options other than remote counseling should be advised of those options. In most cases, telepsychiatry is employed because without it, the patient would not have access to such services, or would not have access to them at a cost he or she could afford. As telemedicine and telemental health continue to achieve mainstream acceptance, however, this will change. Clients will have multiple options for treatment available to them. Many will choose telemental health because they prefer it; several of the studies we have cited herein have at least alluded to this possibility. There will be those clients, however, who are not comfortable receiving treatment remotely, or who prefer the "personal touch" of face-to-face treatment. It falls to the clinician to advise the client of those other options available at the outset of treatment.

Clinicians Should be Creative about how to Approximate Best Practices

Most clinicians today were not originally trained to provide their services through teleconferencing. It is likely that the overwhelming majority of clinicians, from psychiatrists to licensed therapists, et al, received their training in person, face to face with the persons providing it and the individuals whom the clinician treated while learning his or her specialty. Using video teleconferencing can thus provide some unique challenges with regard to best practices. What is the exact etiquette for treating someone over a video link for, say, depression, as opposed to agoraphobia., as opposed to an eating disorder? How does the clinician know to proceed in each unique case when his or her experience of the patient is limited to sound and video connecting him or her to someone many miles away?

As technology continues to advance, more and more virtual reality will be achieved where teleconferencing is concerned. While it may never be the case that a holographic doctor appears like magic in the room to interact with a patient who is, in fact, miles away from a qualified professional, we will see advances in sensing technology and in quality of video and sound that will minimize the limitations of teleconferencing over time. It will still fall to clinicians while this advancement continues, however, to do the best they can. They will at times have to use their imaginations and improvise best practices, based on their education and experience, in order to serve their remote clients.

Conclusion:
Moving Forward One Step
at a Time

Why should your program or facility support telehealth, including teleEAP and telepsychiatry? Simply stated, telepsychiatry is the future of mental healthcare in the United States. It addresses the current and worsening shortage of mental health professionals, it reduces costs and eliminates travel logistics, it helps clients to more quickly develop rapport with providers, and – perhaps most importantly – clients seem actually to *prefer* receiving mental health services remotely.

In a nation where one in twenty Americans lives with a serious mental illness, but far fewer than half of those individuals receive the necessary treatment, we MUST be willing to embrace substantive change in the model of public mental health we are using. The transition away from institutionalized care to community mental health did not solve the problem. While some individuals who would otherwise have lived as virtual prisoners their whole lives did benefit from the community mental health approach, many more affected individuals relapsed, never received needed treatment, wound up homeless, or found themselves wards of the state within the criminal justice system. In many cases, deinstitutionalization has created a vicious cycle in which those who require care do not get it, but they continue to suffer (and their continued suffering produces behavior that keeps them locked in that cycle of suffering).

Unfortunately, even a combined model of hospitals serving as close backup to community mental health facilities cannot solve the worsening problem of mental health in America – a problem that came to the forefront in recent years as the result of high-profile violence from individuals with obvious mental problems who were nonetheless free to act out and harm others. Scandals involving long wait times for veterans seeking healthcare and mental treatment (for PTSD and other mental issues) only exacerbated public outcry. Why, the public asked, were we not *doing something* to address the worsening mental healthcare shortage?

As evidenced by the great successes the VA has had with telemental health solutions, telepsychiatry and teleEAP represent the future of mental healthcare in the United States. They offer a true solution, an innovative means of providing care to those who require it. While the only way to truly solve a shortage of mental healthcare professionals is to provide incentives for more individuals to become mental healthcare professionals, telemental health allows one provider to see more patients more quickly. This acts as a multiplier, bringing care to underserved or physically remote (or even dangerous) locales while also allowing one provider to increase his or her patient load without undue strain on his or her ability to perform those duties.

This book has made the case for telepsychiatry: It is needed because it provides one of the few true solutions to the desperate need for more mental health services in the United States. It works so effectively because it reduces or eliminates travel time, allows for more flexible scheduling, increases patient comfort, and reduces costs. To support telepsychiatry, and to work for the mainstreaming of telep-sychiatry, is to work for the only feasible and rational future of mental healthcare in this nation — a future that sees the overwhelming majority of those who need treatment receiv-ing that treatment. Telepsychiatry succeeds wherever it is applied. Widespread implementation and mainstream acceptance of telepsychiatry (and telehealth in general) must occur in the public and private sectors. While we are taking many steps toward this goal, your continued support of the viability and efficacy of telepsychiatry will go a long way toward convincing lawmakers to remove legal barriers to telemental health services – even as the public in general comes to accept more and more aspects of telehealth technology in their daily lives.

Moving Forward Into a New And Technologically Advanced Future

Telepsychiatry gives providers greater choice of personnel while giving patients greater access to care at lower costs. No, it is not yet the means of choice for mental health practitioners... but we see, even now at the forefront of the field, the first steps towards that goal. Telepsychiatry is more convenient, provides a greater perception of security and confidentiality, and allows fewer providers to serve a broader client base. While regulatory and insurance coverage obstacles remain, the limits to telepsychiatry are no longer defined by the technologies involved. Instead, the expansion and mainstream adoption of telepsychiatry is a matter of informing the public – and creating policies, nationally and industry-wide, that support telepsychiatry's many benefits. You can help the industry achieve that brilliant future by supporting the implementation of telepsychiatry in your own practice, in your own market, in your own field... and in so doing, you can help improve the state of public mental health in the United States.

(Endnotes)

1   http://www.mentalhealth.gov/basics/myths-facts/

2   http://www.nami.org/factsheets/mentalillness_factsheet.pdf

3   https://www.washingtonpost.com/news/wonk/
    wp/2012/12/17/seven-facts-about-americas-mental-health-
    care-system/

4   http://www.uniteforsight.org/mental-health/module2

5   http://www.nationalhomeless.org/factsheets/Mental_Illness.
    pdf

6   https://www.geneticliteracyproject.org/2015/10/13/autism-
    increase-mystery-solved-no-its-not-vaccines-gmos-glypho-
    sate-or-organic-foods/

7   http://bhpr.hrsa.gov/shortage/hpsas/designationcriteria/
    mentalhealthhpsacriteria.html

8   http://mic.com/articles/24564/only-38-of-americans-get-
    mental-health-care-when-they-need-it-and-for-one-simple-
    reason

9   http://www.scientificamerican.com/article/a-neglect-of-
    mental-illness/

10 http://jsahealthmd.com/the-history-of-telemental-health/

11 https://www.e-psychiatry.com/telepsychiatry-case-study.php

12 https://en.wikipedia.org/wiki/Polycom

13 https://en.wikipedia.org/wiki/VSee

14 https://doxyme.freshdesk.com/support/solutions/articles/5000542065-is-doxy-me-hipaa-compliant-

15 http://www.doctorsreview.com/gadgets/free-telemedicine-comes-your-iphone/

16 https://www.healthcarelawtoday.com/2014/08/20/georgia-composite-medical-board-issues-new-telemedicine-rules/

17 http://mobihealthnews.com/48877/does-veterinary-case-point-the-way-to-telemedicines-next-legal-battleground/

18 http://www.bizjournals.com/birmingham/news/2015/11/30/blue-cross-to-start-covering-telemedicine-services.html

19 http://www.americantelemed.org/resources/telemedicine-practice-guidelines/telemedicine-practice-guidelines/practice-guidelines-for-teledermatology#.VpkBgfkrJhE

20 https://www.e-psychiatry.com/telepsychiatry-case-study.php

21 http://www.easna.org/research-and-best-practices/what-is-eap/

22 http://www.ssa.gov/policy/docs/ssb/v65n4/v65n4p3.html

23 http://www.ncbi.nlm.nih.gov/pmc/articles/PMC2426909/

24 http://www.apa.org/monitor/2011/06/telehealth.aspx

25 http://www.businessinsurance.com/article/20141207/NEWS03/312079961?tags=|307|309|70|74

26 https://www.psychologytoday.com/blog/the-act-violence/201402/why-dont-employees-use-eap-services

27 http://telehealth.org/

28 http://onlinetherapyinstitute.com/

29 http://www.ncda.org/aws/NCDA/pt/sd/news_article/89850/_PARENT/layout_details_cc/false

30 http://medical-dictionary.thefreedictionary.com/community+mental+health

31 http://www.euro.who.int/__data/assets/pdf_file/0019/74710/E82976.pdf

32 http://files.eric.ed.gov/fulltext/EJ875402.pdf

33 http://www.teladoc.com

34 http://www.doctorondemand.com/

35 https://amwell.com/

36 https://mdlive.com/

37 http://www.prnewswire.com/news-releases/mdlive-announces-50-million-of-new-funding-300103850.html

38 http://jsahealthmd.com/why-jsa-health/

39 http://forefronttelecare.com/

40 https://www.e-psychiatry.com/

41 http://hitconsultant.net/2015/11/04/genoa-acquires-telepsychiatry-provider-1docway/

42 http://www.ihi.org/engage/initiatives/tripleaim/Pages/default.aspx

43 http://www.ihi.org/engage/initiatives/tripleaim/Pages/default.aspx

44 http://www.ncbi.nlm.nih.gov/pmc/articles/PMC2777553/

45 http://www.bdcadvisors.com/integrating-physical-and-behavioral-health/

46 http://www.ptsd.va.gov/professional/treatment/overview/ptsd-telemental.asp

47 http://www.va.gov/opa/pressrel/pressrelease.cfm?id=2646

48 https://en.wikipedia.org/wiki/Cognitive_behavioral_therapy

49 http://www.ncbi.nlm.nih.gov/pmc/articles/PMC2911004/

50 http://www.jahonline.org/article/S1054-139X(05)00375-7/fulltext?mobileUi=0

51 https://en.wikipedia.org/wiki/Exposure_therapy

52 https://www.1docway.com/blog/2015/7/21/anxiety-disorders-are-underdiagnosed-and-undertreated-in-primary-care

53 http://users.clas.ufl.edu/msscha/psych/pilotstudy_ptsd_telehealth.pdf

54 https://en.wikipedia.org/wiki/Behavior_modification

55 https://www.researchgate.net/profile/Jon_Elhai/publication/5913450_Therapist_adherence_and_competence_with_manualized_cognitive-behavioral_therapy_for_PTSD_delivered_via_videoconferencing_technology/links/02e7e530005e74ed91000000.pdf

56 http://www.ptsd.va.gov/professional/treatment/overview/ptsd-telemental.asp

57 https://en.wikipedia.org/wiki/Motivational_interviewing

58 http://www.trialsjournal.com/content/8/1/18

59 http://europepmc.org/abstract/med/19067501

60 http://www.div12.org/sites/default/files/WhatIsProblemSolvingTherapy.pdf

61 http://europepmc.org/articles/pmc3519946